I0429326

ALCOHOL & ALCOHOLISM

What You Should Know

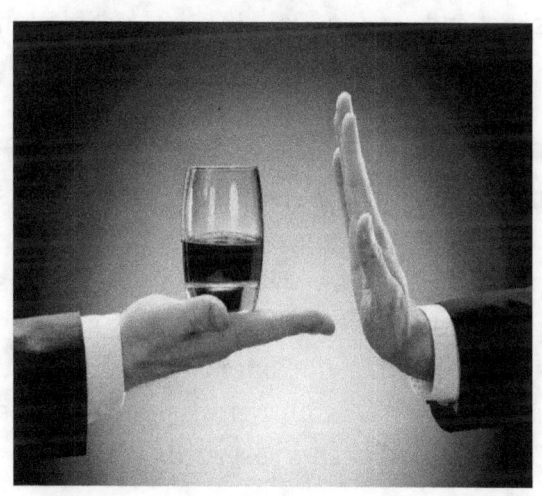

By

Paolo Jose de Luna

Paolo Jose de Luna

otherwise, by any usage or abuse of any policies, processes, or directions contained within is the solitary and utter responsibility of the recipient reader. Under no circumstances will any legal responsibility or blame be held against the publisher for any reparation, damages, or monetary loss due to the information herein, either directly or indirectly.

Respective authors own all copyrights not held by the publisher.

The information herein is offered for informational purposes solely, and is universal as so. The presentation of the information is without contract or any type of guarantee assurance.

The trademarks that are used are without any consent, and the publication of the trademark is without permission or backing by the trademark owner. All trademarks and brands within this book are for clarifying purposes only and are the owned by the owners themselves, not affiliated with this document.

Table of Contents

Introduction

Going out at night for a drink or two is really tempting, right? Definitely! Who can say "no" to hanging out with friends and having some fun? Well... it's just that too much alcohol might just take its toll on you eventually. And by that, it means sooner rather than later. Alcohol is a substance contained in many leisure drinks like beer, vodka, whiskey, rum, scotch, gin – they're all over the place! There are a lot of drinks and beverages that contain alcohol and you just can't stop yourself from enjoying yourself. However, alcohol can also hit your body like a truck in more ways than one.

You're probably no stranger when it comes to alcohol being promoted with the tagline, "Drink moderately". It's true that too much alcohol will mess with you in a lot of ways. You get drunk and messed up, you'll be lucky to even get back to your car. But alcohol is more than just having a little dose of fun. This particular substance hits your health in a lot of ways and most of them aren't good.

There are a lot of people who will voice out the bad of alcohol. Go to any health professional that you know and you can be certain that they'll be telling you that alcohol is bad for your health. Are they just speaking nonsense? Are they just scaring you? Well, these questions might come from someone who blinds himself from the truth. The answers to those questions are out there in the open and all the advices from people around you are there for good reason.

Let me say it to you straight – TOO MUCH ALCOHOL IS BAD FOR YOUR HEALTH.

Sure, you'll be having fun and laughing your heart out with your friends, but in a few years (and for some, it could take only few months) time, you'll be lying on a hospital bed with a busted liver and a pair of dysfunctional kidneys that are damaged beyond repair. By that time, I'm sure that you'll be wallowing in regret and you'll probably be telling yourself, "I shouldn't have drunk that much when I was still young."

Alcohol is considered to be a toxic substance to the body. With the various content of liquor, your body suffers damage through the process of digestion and elimination. You might feel euphoric, but that's just the ethanol, a depressive component in alcohol, talking to you. Little by little, the cells in your liver, stomach, intestines, and even brain are dying from the effects of liquor. Within a few years, you'll be suffering from a myriad of diseases like liver cirrhosis, kidney failure, chronic heart disease, stroke, and even cancer. You've got so much to live for and you're worth more than a stack of beer or a bottle of whiskey.

You have to think about yourself, your family, your friends, your colleagues – everyone that you'll be leaving behind after you've been buried six feet underground because you've been diagnosed with complicated metastatic liver cancer due toexcessive alcohol consumption. The worst part is that it won't be a quick death – you'll be suffering for many weeks, months, or even years from the pain, from the debts, and from the sadness that everyone around you experience as they see you wallowing in guilt, regret, and pain.

The goal of this book is to talk you out of drinking alcohol. Maybe because you're suffering, or maybe because you just need help – that's probably why you got a hand on this book. We'll be talking about the hard facts and truths on alcohol, its effects on your health, and how you can stand back up and defeat the addiction that ties you and your life down to stupor.

Chapter 1 - The Hidden Truths of Alcohol

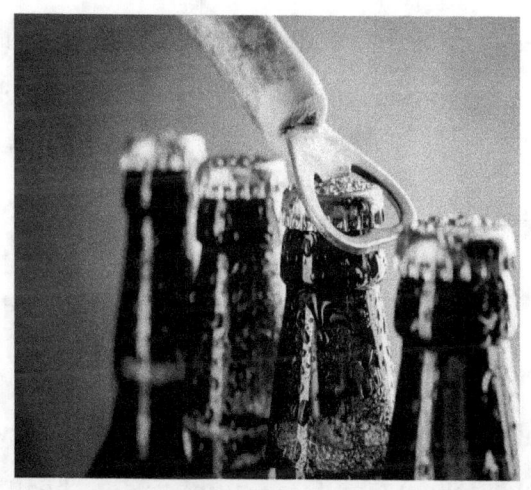

The term "alcohol" bears similar semblance to the word "liquor" as the two can be used interchangeably due to their meanings. However, the two should be differentiated in a sense that they are quite diverse when you look at them deeper. Alcohol, or specifically *ethanol*, is a substance found in alcoholic beverages or liquor. Ethanol is considered to be a psychoactive drug as it causes depression to the nervous system. Low doses of this substance causes euphoria or a sense of elation, decreased anxiety, and improved social interactions. However, too much ethanol in the body can lead to intoxication or getting drunk, lethargy, and even unconsciousness. Chronic consumption of alcohol is never considered a healthy habit which leads to alcohol abuse, alcoholic dependency, alcoholism, and a number of health problems which includes cancer, liver cirrhosis, gastrointestinal diseases, and more.

While liquor gives you a sense of accomplishment, this only lasts for a short time. From the hangover that you get, you'll be suffering from excruciating headaches that can last from a few hours up to a couple of days. You'll only get relief after taking a healthy dose of anti-hangover remedies that is quite personal to each individual. While one person may eat a smorgasbord of a breakfast to cure his hangover, another one might need a cup of coffee to fight off the headache. Regardless of your remedy, a hangover is something you definitely don't want to have, especially if you've got chores, work, or school on the following day.

What hurts is that though the "happiness" that liquor gives you is only temporary, everything else becomes "permanent" in the long run if you're not careful. This includes the various effects on your health, the psychological effects of alcohol on your brain, and the social impact that it brings into your daily life. It's because of these that a lot of people tell you that resorting to alcohol is never going to be good when it comes to solving your problems.

The Commercialization of Liquor

Once in your lifetime, you've probably seen at least one or two commercials about liquor. There's a pattern when it comes down to advertising something like alcohol and it's a pattern that you'll be surprised no matter how much you dive into it. Have you ever noticed how sexualized most liquor commercials are? Well, that's the thing about it – liquor advertisements need to be overly sexual or presented as socially acceptable to attract potential customers. You've probably seen a sexy and voluptuous girl drinking a particular brand of beer or whiskey in a bar. If not, you've probably seen a commercial where a guy goes to a bar or somewhere similar and "coincidentally" picks up a hot girl after drinking that particular brand of liquor.

These types of commercials easily catch the attention of people, regardless of the kind of product. Also notice how the liquor appears in the later part of the advertisement as it serves as the lasting impression of the commercial. You remember most of the details of the commercial, but the one thing that you're left remembering the most is the last scene with the beer or whiskey or whatever kind of liquor the commercial may be advertising.

And then notice the last segment of the commercial where it flashes a black screen with white text that says, "Drink Moderately", or something similar along those lines. It appears for a second or even half a second for most commercials. And even with just these few words, they hold the hard fact about alcohol – it isn't good for you especially if taken excessively.

The big companies make billions of dollars every year with the production of liquor. With the many variants to choose from, it's no wonder that a lot of people tend to buy alcohol, sometimes without even knowing it. But the most common places where you can get liquor are from bars, liquor stores, and clubs. However, the sad fact is that you can easily buy liquor in convenience stores now. It's through this easy method that many fall into temptation and resort to chronic alcoholism.

The bottom line is alcohol is not and will never be good for your health. If you've been drinking liquor and constantly defend yourself with the various "health benefits" that alcohol brings, it's just drinking in small amounts. But if you're drinking yourself out with several bottles every night, then that's a whole different story. If that's the case, you should expect to be greeted with soon-to-be longtime buddies like cancer, liver cirrhosis, heart problems, pancreatitis, and a lot more.

Laws Regarding Liquor

There are laws regulating the buying and selling of alcohol around the world. This covers the manufacturing, selling, and consuming any type of alcoholic beverage which can subject a person or a company to pay damages indicated by the law. The laws on alcohol aim to reduce the health risks and the social effects that alcohol consumption causes.

The laws regulate the selling of alcoholic beverages below the legal drinking age which can be as low as 16 years old up to 25 years old and can also depend on the type of liquor. While there are some countries that don't have a legal age for alcohol consumption, most have it at 18 years of age. Stores that sell liquor need to have licenses that prove they are allowed and credited retailers of alcoholic products and they often come with taxes that add up to the cost of alcohol. Without getting licensed, stores may receive a penalty that they need to pay off with cash or they may even be subject to closure or have the owner imprisoned for a set number of months for disobeying the law. There are also cases wherein consuming liquor is completely banned due to a number of reasons which may include religious beliefs, public health, or public safety.

But the reality now is that many stores – most stores – nowadays don't even check for the legal drinking age of those who buy alcohol. Oftentimes, clerks will just "judge" if the person buying alcohol is of legal age just by looking. Regulations indicate that those who buy liquor need to present their valid IDs with pictures. This assures the identity of the customer is of legal drinking age.

But the alcohol laws has a loop hole in it that many seem to overlook. Though the customer may be of legal drinking age, he can bring the alcoholic beverages on private property and allow minors to drink liquor. This clearly breaks the laws set on the standards and regulations on alcohol consumption, but once it's on private property, no one has the capability to watch everything that transpires. In this regard, parents should be responsible in guiding their children about alcohol consumption.

Chapter 2 - The Effects of Alcohol on Health

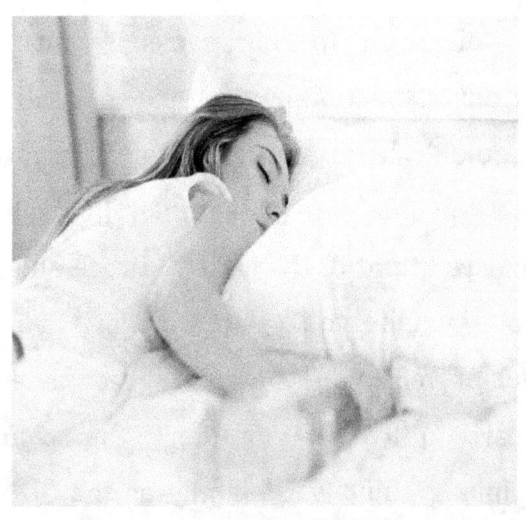

Now let's get down to business. Health is a very common topic to discuss when it comes to alcohol. As mentioned in the introduction of this book, we're here to talk you out in drinking alcohol. It's not just for a week, it's not just for a couple of months – what we want is for you to stop drinking liquor altogether and stop being dependent on it.

If you want to talk someone out of drinking, mentioning the topic on "health" shouldn't be exempted. That's because most people care about their lives and they're afraid of dying. If you care about your own life, you'd start worrying if your doctor tells you you've only got a few years to live. If you don't, then start thinking about your family as they'll be the ones suffering from your loss.

This book will present you with the cold, hard facts and I'll tell you now that things aren't going to be pretty. I'll be frank, direct, and straight to the point. Sure, you might be terrified, but if it gets you out of your drinking habit, that's just peachy.

Here are the things that you need to know how alcohol can sabotage your health:

The Heart and Cardiovascular System

The heart is one of the vital organs affected by chronic alcoholism. If you drink too much for too long, it can damage the cardiac tissues, leading to a number of cardiovascular problems which can include cardiomyopathy, myocardial infarction, cardiac arrhythmia, cardiovascular disease, atherosclerosis, and hypertension.

Alcohol weakens the binding of the cardiac muscles, leading to a weak heart and can later on develop in congestive heart failure. The blood vessels also suffer from alcohol because the vessel structures weaken, leading to the development of stroke, aneurysm formation, aneurysm rupture, and arterial or venous diseases.

Drinking too much alcohol also leads to an increase in the levels of triglycerides or fats in the blood. This leads to a pyramid of diseases that come from the rise in serum triglycerides which include high blood pressure, myocardial infarction, and stroke. Because many alcoholic drinks are rich in calories, it can also contribute to obesity. There are even some reported cases where some have suffered a heart attack or a stroke because of binge drinking.

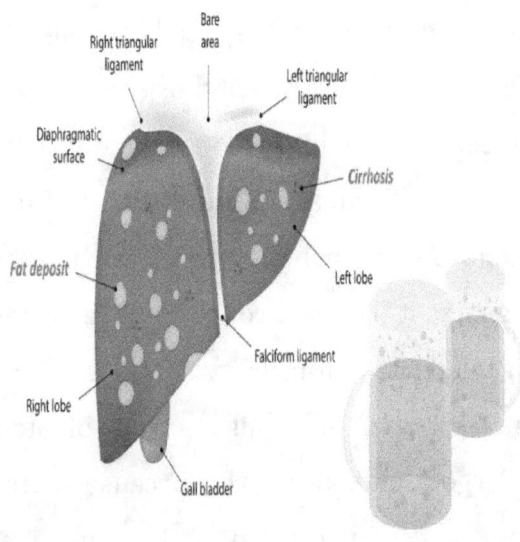

The Liver

If we're talking about alcohol and its effects on health, the liver is the topmost reason of discussion about that. The liver is an organ that serves as a "filter" to everything that we eat and drink – including liquor. When the liver filters too much waste and the waste is retained in the liver, the liver slowly gets damaged overtime which can lead to health problems like liver cirrhosis and liver cancer. For many alcoholics, the liver suffers the most because the various chemicals in alcoholic drinks damage the organ as it passes through the liver when digested. In autopsies, you can see that the liver of an alcoholic becomes bloated, enlarged, and discolored because of the damage compared to a healthy liver which is shiny, smooth, and firm.

Fatty liver results from the damage occurring to the liver cells. The enlargement of the liver results in the malfunction of the organ, resulting in a high level of waste products defined by the urea and nitrogen in the blood. Creatinine in the blood which indicates the normal fluid excretion in the body also rises when the liver is damaged. Overtime, the fluid exchange in the tissues also malfunction since the liver is the one supposed to do that by maintaining a normal level of albumin in the blood. This results in the swelling of the abdomen due to fluids pooling in the peritoneal cavity. Fluids also pool in the legs which result in large, elephant-like legs that indicate fluid overload. If the kidneys get affected, you may even notice a drastic decline in your urine, indicating that the fluids in your body are not properly excreted.

The treatment for liver disease isn't pretty either. Treating liver infections like hepatitis involves the use of antibiotics, vitamins, and therapeutics drugs that are administered via an intravenous line that goes through your veins. These medications are often painful physically and painful financially as they are expensive. But they're necessary if you want your liver to live.

For more serious conditions like liver cirrhosis which often results in severe abdominal bloating, a paracentesis needs to be done. This involves the use of a large-bore needle inserted into the peritoneal cavity to drain the fluid that pooled up in the abdomen. For those who have liver cancer, a surgery may be necessary to excise the cancerous tissues from the liver. Chemotherapy is often done after surgery to inhibit the metastatic growth of the cancer. However, many cases of liver cirrhosis and liver cancer don't have good prognoses because of the severity of the disease. The liver bears a crucial role in the body and if it gets damaged, it's just a matter of time that you suffer from its effects.

The Pancreas

The pancreas is the organ situated just near the liver. Though smaller in size, it still has a vital function which maintains the body's health. Excessive consumption of alcohol leads to the damage of the pancreas. This leads to the pancreas to produce toxic substances that lead to inflammation which is termed as pancreatitis – a life-threatening inflammation of the pancreas that prevents the proper digestion of food. Pancreatitis is painful and may require both medical management and surgery to repair the damaged pancreas. The scary fact is that pancreatitis has a high mortality rate because of the potential buildup of toxic substances in the pancreas, later spilling into the peritoneal cavity. This often leads to sudden death even when asleep.

Alcoholics are also prone to develop diabetes mellitus because the pancreas also regulates the production of insulin – a substance that regulates blood sugar. With not enough insulin or not having enough sensitivity to insulin, the blood sugar rises and leads to a number of diseases like high blood pressure, buildup of waste products in the blood, a weakened immune system, and nonhealing wounds that often result in a limb being amputated or cut off.

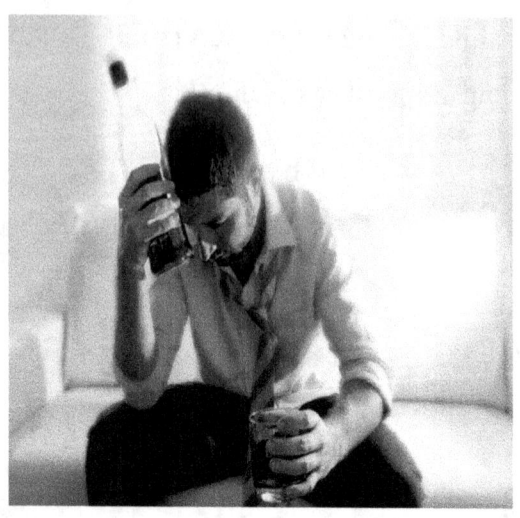

Other Health Problems

There are a lot more health problems that we can talk about when it comes to alcohol. Fetal alcohol syndrome can result from an alcoholic mother which is a group of signs and symptoms that result in the stunted growth of an infant. Chronic alcoholism can also result in impotence and reproductive problems for both men and women. Consuming alcohol on a daily basis also leads to the damage of the nervous system which leads to poor balance and coordination, poor short-term memory, decreased attention span, inability to concentrate, and more.

We could take hours if we keep on talking about the effects of alcohol on your health. But the bottom line is that you'll be the one suffering from all of these health problems if you don't stop. Drinking, drinking liquor that is, is never and will never be good for you.

Chapter 3 - Recovering from Alcoholism

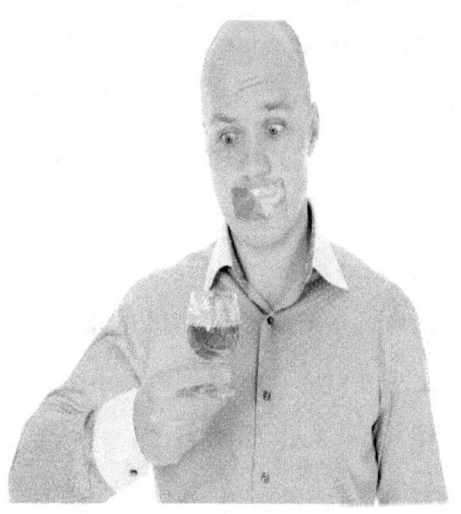

Stopping from drinking altogether may be easier said than done. Let's face it, it's never going to be easy, especially if you've been drinking yourself for years. Are you doing something wrong with your life right now? YES. Is it too late to make that change? Definitely **NO**.

Whatever it is that you're thinking, it's never too late to step up and make that change. If you want to stop drinking, there are things that you can do to recover from the horrible habit of drinking. Here are the steps that you need to take to make the new start that you need in your life:

Committing Yourself

If you want to start the change that your life needs, you have to make that commitment that you really want to stop drinking. Have a look yourself in the mirror and tell that person in front of you, "You're going to stop drinking. You're strong, you're smart, you're persistent – I know that you can do it. I believe in you." The first step in every goal you have to

make   is   to   commit   yourself
wholeheartedly without any hesitation.

Setting Goals and Weighing Pros/Cons

To make things more realistic, you should make a goal if you want to stop drinking. Set an attainable goal. You can have a week without drinking, then going for a month, then for three months, then for half a year, then for a year. All of this will just let you grow more as a person and your resistance to alcohol will just build. The longer that you shy away from alcohol, the better your life will become.

Weighing the risks and the benefits will also help you in recovering from alcoholism. Think about this: the average price of a beer in the US is about $5 and you drink about two to three bottles of beer everyday. You just saved $100 in just a week! You can buy more important and more awesome things with that cash like a new game for your Xbox, a new office chair, or even bags filled with groceries that might last you for a week!

The Healing Process

The abrupt stopping of drinking alcohol may not be for everyone. There's a thing that we call "withdrawal" which arise when you suddenly stop drinking liquor. Getting help from your doctor is important so that you can get sober safely and gradually. It may involve the use of medications that help in relieving the signs and symptoms of withdrawal, as well as diverting your attention from triggers of attacks like eating chocolates, reading a book, and more productive activities.

Finding a New Purpose

When you've committed yourself to rehabilitation, you need to find a new meaning in life so you can live out the new ideals that you've built up and the things that you've learned. You have to make sure to take care of yourself both physically and emotionally, eating right and including exercise in your daily activities. Build healthy relationships with friends and family so you get a strong support system for your battle against alcoholism. Start developing new hobbies and interests so you can divert your attention away from drinking and doing more productive and meaningful things in life. The possibilities are just endless when you stop drinking. You save more money, you save more time, and you promote your health to its maximum capacity. The best thing about it is that you'll feel all the good in shying away from alcohol in just a few weeks.

Getting a Support System

Lastly, having a strong bond with your friends and family is important if you want to succeed in your recovery from being dependent on alcohol. You need people who believe in you and who help you whenever you need a push. You need to have people who encourage you to pursue your goals and support you when the time warrants it. But the strongest factor to this support system is yourself – you need to believe in yourself that you can do it and you can stop drinking once and for all.

Chapter 4 - Liquor and Criminal Acts

Alcohol and the law often get tangled together in a conversation. That's because liquor is a prime suspect in substance abuse of many people. Though defended as being only a "drink", alcohol is considered as a harmful substance that should be controlled and regulated by the law. If given to minors, it can cause a myriad of problems later in their lives like substance abuse, alcohol dependence, vehicular accidents, and even resorting to violent crimes.

Drunk driving is one of the most common cases of liquor involved in criminal acts. Those who get drunk and then drive are often the cause for deadly accidents that claim the lives of not just the driver, but also innocent pedestrians that are just minding their own business. Each year, hundreds and thousands of lives are taken by cases of drunk driving. Oftentimes, the victims are just innocent bystanders subjected to the idiocy that those who drink and drive kill. Today, driving under the influence, even without any other criminal record, will be subjected to punishment if found to be guilty of being drunk while driving. Police officers nowadays carry a breath analyzer which detects the presence of ethanol, the substance in liquor, to prove someone has been drinking. Punishment for drunk driving alone can range from a few days to months in prison depending on the country's laws. But at times, drunk driving is usually paired with other charges like homicide, murder, damage to public property, damage to private property, disturbance of the peace, and more.

Being drunk also accounts for charges involved in sexual assaults. There are thousands to millions of cases worldwide that indicate those who committed sexual crimes like sexual harassment, rape, sexual assault, and more have been drinking. There are even cases wherein women have been purposely drunk by a man or a group of men and then bring the woman to a private property then proceed to rape the woman while unconscious. Usual locations for these crimes are often bars, nightclubs, hotels, and private residences.

Because alcohol is a legal substance, it is the cause of most violent crimes which include assault, child abuse, and spousal abuse. You often hear children telling stories of their drunkard fathers or wives telling their horrifying experiences of having a drunkard husband. Those who rely on alcohol too much are found to commit violence towards their spouse or children as a form of defense mechanism. This also hurts their social relationships with other people as they become more focused on getting the drink rather than building a healthy relationship with people. About 33% of victims that were attacked by their spouse or boyfriend or girlfriend reported that their partner had been drink. About 31% of victims reported that they were attacked by strangers who have been drunk. Almost all of the reports on family violence also include alcohol as some cases of violence between acquaintances have been connected to alcohol.

Alcoholism is often connected with the use of drugs. Heroin, cocaine, marijuana – you name it, you can never have a person who uses drugs to never drink alcohol. Studies have found that about 70% to 80% of illegal drug users are also alcoholics. Because of the interaction of both drugs and alcohol, this can lead a person to do heinous crimes of violence ranging from assault, sexual harassment, and public disturbance to homicide, murder, and rape. It's already a given that illegal drug use will result in the arrest and punishment of a person, but pairing it up with drinking alcohol just make things worse. Furthermore, the health risks that alcohol does to the body is further exacerbated because of drugs and vice-versa. You don't have to be surprised to see a drug user suffering from a heart disease or liver cancer while in their late 20s or 30s.

Getting drunk and committing a crime isn't that far off. You'll see a number of cases on TV or in social media wherein people have been arrested by the police because of being under the influence of alcohol. Either by drunk driving up to more serious crimes like murder or rape, alcohol has never disappeared in the spotlight. Liquor blurs your senses and alters your consciousness, leading you to act through your inhibitions. May it be hurting someone you never meant to but you've only been think about or sexually assaulting a woman who you thought was beautiful, these will become crimes if you let alcohol take control of you.

Believe me – it's not fun to stay in prison even for just a couple of hours. Having been incarcerated and getting to put on your records that you've been arrested or you've been to jail once will give you a hard time building social relationships, traveling, or even getting a decent job.

And it's not just about yourself, you also have to think about your family. If you get arrested for something like drunk driving, who will be the one providing for your spouse and child at home? Who will be watching your son's baseball game during parents' day? Who will be the raising your family? Will you let your family suffer from your absence because of one stupid mistake of letting alcohol take control of you? Think about it.

Conclusion

Alcoholism is one of the most common problems in the world right now. It affects our health, not just physically, but emotionally and socially as well. The body suffers from a number of health problems which include liver cirrhosis, cancer, cardiovascular disease, pancreatitis, and a whole lot more. Aside from the physical toll that it causes to our body, the emotional turmoil that we experience from being dependent on liquor is terrible. You become moody and you can never tell what you're going to do once your consciousness becomes blurry. You might commit a crime like driving while drunk or even hurting someone you didn't even mean to. But the regret is useless when you've already done the crime and you'll spend many years in prison all for a stupid mistake that you could have avoided in the first place.

The road to recovery for an alcoholic is never easy – nothing ever is. It will take time, it will take effort, but most of all, it will take patience. You can't just say, "I'll stop drinking tomorrow!" and just grab a beer by the following night. You need to be committed to this goal and you're going to need help. There are a lot of ways that you can do to stop drinking and you need the help of the important people in your life to do it – including yourself.

So believe in yourself and stop drinking. You can do it and better start NOW!